VALSARTÁN

Dr. Frank C. Quimby

Genuine viability of valsartan on hypertension and absolute cardiovascular gamble: survey and ramifications of a translational examination program

Dynamic

The pharmacological viability of different monotherapy, single pill, and mix treatments of the angiotensin II receptor blocker valsartan have been laid out, predominantly through randomized controlled preliminaries that utilized comparative systemic and factual stages and subsequently empowered union of proof. This present reality viability of valsartan has been concentrated widely, however the overall absence of logical and specialized compatibility of these investigations render blend basically unimaginable. Until now, all have zeroed in on circulatory strain results, regardless of proof based calls to grade antihypertensive treatment to patients' complete cardiovascular gamble. Seven studies from a T3 translational research program on valsartan monotherapy, single pill combinations, and the factors that influence blood pressure and total cardiovascular risk outcomes are examined. Every one of the seven investigations inspected not just the effect of valsartan-put together regimens with respect to pulse values and control, yet additionally, inside a measurable various leveled approach, the doctor and patient-related determinants of these circulatory strain results. Two examinations likewise explored the determinants and results of valsartan-put together treatment with respect to add up to cardiovascular gamble - among the main investigations to involve this hazard coefficient as a result as opposed to just a determinant. These seven examinations incorporated a sum of 19,533 patients, contributed by 3434 doctor specialists in Belgium - a nation especially appropriate for observational viability studies in light of socioeconomics and the study of disease transmission. Each study utilized a similar systemic and measurable stage. We sum up the effect of different valsartan regimens on such results as circulatory strain values and control, change altogether cardiovascular gamble, and decrease in risk by somewhere around one class. We likewise survey the consequences of factual staggered and strategic demonstrating of doctor and patient-related determinants on these results, including the extent of change owing to a doctor class impact before patients enter the condition. In its various details, valsartan has significant true advantages in bringing down pulse and complete cardiovascular gamble inside a 90-day time span. It is fundamental to comprehend the doctor and patient-related determinants of pulse and complete cardiovascular gamble results related with valsartan treatment. Antihypertensive exploration ought to grow its authentic spotlight on bringing down pulse with an accentuation on bringing down complete cardiovascular examination.

Presentation

Valsartan is an antihypertensive specialist of the class of angiotension II receptor blockers (ARB). These specialists block the angiotensin II sort 1 (AT1) receptor through all pathways, in addition to the renin-angiotensin-aldosterone pathway repressed by angiotensin-changing over catalyst (Expert) inhibitors. Obstructing the AT1 receptor intervenes the pulse (BP) lifting impacts of angiotensin, including vasoconstriction, arrival of aldosterone and antidiuretic chemical, thoughtful enactment, and choking of the efferent glomerular arterioles. Further, by not impeding the angiotensin II sort 2 (AT2) receptor, the gainful impacts of feeling of the AT2 receptor are kept up with, including vasodilation, tissue fix, and cell development restraint.

A few articles offer brilliant surveys of randomized controlled preliminaries (RCTs) on the viability of valsartan. Valsartan has been shown to lower blood pressure in a variety of patient groups, including children, the elderly, and women; patients with diabetes, chronic kidney disease, and cardiovascular disease at high risk; what's more, across racial and ethnic gatherings. Notwithstanding its antihypertensive impact, valsartan has likewise been displayed to make a cardioprotective difference. Treatment with valsartan lessens cardiovascular bleakness and mortality following myocardial infarct (MI) in patients with cardiovascular breakdown and in patients with coronary supply route illness it additionally brings down the frequency of cerebrovascular mishaps. Similar to other ARBs, Valsartan can lower levels of high-sensitivity C-reactive protein and oxidized low-density lipoprotein, two biomarkers of endothelial dysfunction and cardiovascular risk, in the bloodstream. Valsartan has a renoprotective impact in patients with diabetes as well as persistent kidney sickness as recorded by decreased urinary egg whites and protein discharge. In high-risk hypertensive patients, including those with impaired glucose tolerance, diabetes, metabolic syndrome, and obesity, valsartan safeguards metabolic function. Besides, valsartan is protected and very much endured both in mono-and mix treatment and in a wide scope of hypertensive patients.

The focus and justification of the review In this piece, we build on the extensive body of literature on valsartan's effectiveness. We do as such, neither by giving one more survey of adequacy results nor by attempting to give the principal audit of the significantly more noteworthy number of observational examinations on the viability of valsartan in routine clinical practice. An underlying audit of the collection of observational examinations shows extraordinary changeability in the degree and the nature of goals, philosophy, examination, and results;7 the disparate discoveries are probably not going to be illustrative of valsartan's adequacy in the day to day clinical setting.

All things considered, we have decided to survey a novel 'T3' translational (practice-based) research program8 on the viability of valsartan in reality setting. This program includes seven examinations, directed starting around 2004, on different details of valsartan on a sum of 19,533 patients contributed by 7043 doctor specialists in Belgium - a nation especially appropriate for observational viability studies as a result of the strategic benefits of a little yet thickly populated country with two significant societies and dialects, as well as metropolitan and provincial regions. Our examination program utilizes a coordinated system for observational viability issues in which the (regular) question of whether valsartan works in routine clinical practice is supplemented by a few extra inquiries to acquire a thorough comprehension of the clinical elements of valsartan-based regimens in the administration of hypertension.

In addition, our research program was one of the first in the health sciences to employ social science-derived methodological and statistical techniques to examine the extent to which physician-related factors influence valsartan treatment outcomes prior to patient-related factors. Patients seen by a similar clinician are presented to his/her hypertension information, experience, and practice designs. Technically, this goes against the assumption that observations are statistically independent. Despite the fact that there is evidence of potential physician determinants, previous studies have not statistically accounted for the potential class effect of multiple patients being treated by the same physician-investigator. In this manner, both patient-and doctor related factors should be analyzed to all the more likely comprehend the changeability in BP results in day to day clinical practice and any distinctions in RCT viability versus 'genuine world' adequacy.

A last clever component of our examination program, carried out in two ongoing examinations, is the utilization of all out cardiovascular gamble (TCVR) as a result mark of antihypertensive treatment with valsartan. The 2007 European Culture of Cardiology-European Culture of Hypertension (ESC-ESH) Rules and the 2009 ESH rule reappraisal suggest that TCVR be evaluated methodiaclly in all patients with blood vessel hypertension and that the force of antihypertensive administration be reviewed as a component of TCVR. This appraisal should be possible based on the SCORE models that gauge patients' 10-year chance of lethal CV infection for high and generally safe European nations. Regularly, concentrates on use TCVR (or components thereof) as a determinant or covariate of BP results when, seemingly, TCVR can be utilized as a result variable of the viability of antihypertensive treatment.

From viability to adequacy

Viability alludes to how a treatment functions in ideal conditions, when given to chosen patients by suppliers generally talented at giving it. Interestingly, viability alludes to how a treatment functions under common and variable circumstances, recommended by authorized clinicians with shifting levels of skill and rehearsing across the range of medical services settings, to treat a heterogeneity of patients.

To get the most flawless conceivable adequacy signal, randomized controlled preliminaries will generally be specific in the patients enlisted ('completely sick') and the examiners and focuses taking part in the preliminaries (famous and trusted for their logical characteristics). Treatment is characterized barely by convention and offers little scope for deviation. Clinician-investigators receive thorough instruction on how to identify and treat patients who join the trial. Patients are observed intently during treatment periods that will quite often be short. Treatment is free to patients.

This is both fitting and fundamental for distinguishing an adequacy signal that illustrates, as unambiguously as could really be expected, the pharmacotherapeutic advantage of a specialist under states of ideal control of potential (known and obscure) confounders. However, RCT conditions are not representative of the clinical context in which these agents may be used after receiving marketing approval, and this is especially true for treatments for chronic diseases like hypertension. As a matter of fact, RCTs for drug enlistment purposes look similar to this present reallty setting of everyday clinical practice. Patients range in age, have a variety of comorbidities, come from a variety of socioeconomic backgrounds, and have complicated personal and family medical histories. They are probably not going to get the direction and observing given to subjects in RCTs. The expense of treatment is somewhat theirs. Clinicians, going from amateur to master, accepted their clinical preparation from establishments and offices across the quality range, and may have performed above or underneath the middle of their schooling and preparing associates. Not many offices will match the logical accreditations of those utilized in the enrollment preliminaries.

It isn't is actually to be expected, then, at that point, that this present reality viability of antihypertensive specialists in lessening BP and accomplishing rule suggested targets might vary from the adequacy seen in RCTs. Patients' risk of target organ damage and cardiovascular and renal disease may rise if BP targets are not met. BP results have been connected to patient-related factors, for example, sociodemographics, heritability, history, comorbid conditions, way of life, information about illness and treatment, and drug adherence. The noticed variety in doctors' information about antihypertensive treatment has not been connected straightforwardly to BP results, however it is realized that more seasoned doctors have less authentic information and are less inclined to stick to the guidelines of care while treating hypertension. Additionally, there is evidence that BP outcomes are correlated with physician practice patterns.

RCTs are recommended for determining pharmacological agents' efficacy. Integrated framework for observational effectiveness studies In any case, by need RCTs are compelled as far as patients and clinicians included, and medicines should be restricted to the specialist being scrutinized so that unconfounded surmisings about a specialist's viability can be drawn. Observational investigations are expected to inspect the viability of medications recently recorded to be solid. The majority of observational studies narrowly focus on assessing a treatment's efficacy in "real-world" conditions, leaving important questions unanswered. Whether or not 'the treatment works?', while basic, doesn't resolve the similarly significant inquiries of 'when accomplishes the treatment work, and when not?', ' in whom accomplishes the treatment work, and in whom not?', ' for what reason accomplishes the treatment work in certain patients yet not in others?', ' for what reason does the treatment work for certain clinicians however not with others?', also 'for what reason is the treatment endured by certain patients yet not by others?'

In order to guarantee clinical relevance, scientific value, and technical merit, we have developed an integrated framework for observational studies that has evolved into a de facto quality model. It presents a flowchart of the system utilized in our examination program. Driven by a potential viability adequacy hole in ARB treatment - regardless of the accessibility of proof based practice rules for the administration of hypertension - the structure incorporates four logical objectives operationalized into seven examination steps.

The principal objective is to decide the fluctuation in BP values, BP control, and the leftover TCVR after treatment with a valsartan-based routine. As a result, the first step looks at the observed BP values to see if the hypertension has gone down and if the BP is now within the normal range. In more recent times, step 1 also looks at the extent to which lower BP has reduced TCVR.

The subsequent objective investigates the determinants of noticed pulse decrease at both the doctor and the patient-level. At the doctor level, we assess their insight into hypertension the executives, specifically as depicted in proof based practice rules. We inspect the degree to which they practice comparative with these rules (stage 2). We likewise gather segment and expert information.

At the patient level, we evaluate whether patients stuck to their recommended routine (stage 3). Rather than endeavoring to evaluate adherence with 'pinpoint' precision, we advocate the utilization of brief estimates that can be coordinated effectively into routine clinical practice. These actions may not give the 'genuine' level of a patient's adherence, yet we don't really accept that this is fundamental. Clinicians lack the capacity to deal with broad adherence appraisal. Short and simple techniques that give them an impression regarding whether treatment adherence is an issue in a given patient have been demonstrated to be exceptionally prescient of the gamble for unfortunate treatment reaction and uncontrolled BP. We likewise gather information connected with socioeconomics, clinical status, and information.

The purpose of Step 4 is to create a heuristic profile of the patient's susceptibility to unsuccessful treatment. Deterministic calculations to decide cardiovascular results are accessible (eg, SCORE, Framingham) however are only here and there utilized in essential consideration. Time constraints and a lack of integration with the clinical flow of primary care encounters are two reasons. Clinicians will quite often see deterministic models as prescriptive and limiting their clinical ability in assessing patients and surveying risk. Like adherence appraisal, clinicians favor clinically instinctive direction for distinguishing patients who might be less inclined to accomplish great treatment results.

The third objective is to demonstrate BP results and changes in TCVR. Hierarchical linear regression (step 5) and logistic regression (step 6) are used to accomplish this. Various leveled alludes to measurable techniques in which the class impact on results is assessed before genuine results are determined; in our examination program, the impact of the class of doctor as every one of them contributed a few patients to a review and the following loss of freedom of perception.

Simultaneously, the extent of change in BP results related owing to the treating doctor is assessed. In sync 6, calculated relapse techniques are applied to distinguish autonomous indicators of why a few patients don't answer antihypertensive treatment with valsartan.

The last objective worries proceeded pharmaco-cautiousness. Observational examinations will generally have bigger patient examples than RCTs. This adds factual capacity to the capacity to distinguish wellbeing signals that might not have been identified in earlier RCTs. In this manner observational viability, joined with other post-endorsement exercises, offer a basic supplement to RCTs to identify low-recurrence unfriendly occasions with a genuinely low probability of being recognized in viability preliminaries.

Audit of studies

The examination program involves seven investigations on different valsartan regimens led somewhere in the range of 2004 and 2009: See,

IMPROVE, ADVANCE, Demand, eNOVA, BSCORE, and Astounding. It sums up the examinations concerning year of commencement, evaluable examples, and key patient socioeconomics and valsartan plans included. Studies were started somewhere in the range of 2004 and 2008, with the final remaining one (Fantastic) finished in 2009. Throughout the span of the program, all endorsed monotherapy and (single-pill) blend details were examined, except for valsartan 320 mg. A sum of 19,533 evaluable patients was contributed by 3434 doctor examiners. Five investigations included above and beyond 3000 patients each. Mean (±SD) age was reliable across studies, and the weighted normal was 63.6 years. There were minor changes in orientation appropriation across studies, however on normal orientation was similarly circulated. Overall, somewhat under a fourth of patients were diabetic.

Center goals

Steady with the center targets across the seven investigations were to:

- Evaluate systolic (SBP) and diastolic (DBP) pulse and BP control at 90 days in patients getting a valsartan routine as second-line treatment since first-line treatment fizzled or was not endured;
- Decide the level of difference in BP values at 90 days owing to a doctor class impact;
- Analyze the various leveled (patients 'settled' under doctors) determinants of BP values at 90 days; and discover independent predictors of non-responding to valsartan-focused treatment.

Likewise, the BSCORE and Incredible investigations additionally meant to:

- Evaluate remaining TCVR at 90 days, as well as the extent of patients who accomplished a decrease in TCVR of no less than one classification;
- Decide the level of difference in remaining TCVR at 90 days owing to a doctor class impact;
- Look at the various leveled determinants of remaining TCVR at 90 days; what's more,

- Recognize free indicators of accomplishing an improvement in TCVR of somewhere around one class.

Center procedure

Configuration all reviews incorporated a pattern evaluation at the time that treatment with valsartan was started, and a subsequent appraisal roughly 90 days after the fact. The choice to treat with valsartan was made by the endorsing doctor in light of his/her best clinical judgment. Being an observational review, there were no necessary tests and all information gathered were as accessible from routine clinical practice.

All reviews followed the Statement of Helsinki. In accordance with Belgian laws and regulations as well as directives from the European Union regarding the use of human subjects, approvals were obtained from appropriate ethical committees. All subjects gave informed assent.

Examining Qualified for support in any of the examinations were male and female patients whose treating doctor chose freely and per best clinical judgment to recommend valsartan as second-line mono-or polytherapy, incorporating single-pill mixes with hydrochlorothiazide (HCTZ) or amlodipine. Patients must be hypertensive, characterized as DBP ≥ 90 mmHg (≥80 mmHg for diabetic patients) or potentially SBP ≥ 140 mmHg (≥130 mmHg for diabetic patients). Patients with controlled SBP or potentially DBP at gauge were qualified in the event that the change to a valsartan routine happened in light of the fact that earlier line treatment was not endured. Patients with aversions to any ARBs, thiazides, or calcium channel blockers were rejected; as were patients on any investigational drug in the 30 days before enrolment, and patients endorsed different ARBs during the review time frame.

Factors and estimations

The examinations included just quiet information gathered regularly in clinical practice. The center information model was created based on writing survey and clinical experience. However there were periodic minor varieties across the seven examinations as far as information components included, basically all reviews gathered thoughtfully as well as functionally similar information. All information models are accessible from the comparing creator.

Center information model Doctor survey: practice type, area/setting, patient blend; demographics; wellsprings of data and information connected with hypertension; self-detailed hypertension the board rehearses; remedy designs; controlling side effects; SBP/DBP edges for therapy commencement and strengthening; impression of patient adherence; and familiarity with practice guidelines

Patient standard information: demographics; anthropometrics; hypertension and CV history; comorbidities; lifestyle; earlier antihypertensive drugs; SBP and DBP; doctor announced TCVR (BSCORE and Superb examinations as it were); clinical status; beginning doses; all corresponding enemy of hypertensive and other applicable drugs (recommended according to doctors' clinical judgment); self-revealed and doctor evaluated (0-100) visual simple scale adherence inside the beyond about a month; what's more, adherence and non-adherence ways of behaving.

Patient subsequent information (90 days): SBP and DBP; lingering doctor revealed TCVR (BSCORE and Fantastic examinations as it were); clinical status; changes in dosing since past visit; attending medication(s) taken or changed since past visit (endorsed according to doctors' clinical judgment); self-revealed and doctor appraised adherence inside the beyond 4 weeks (0-100 visual simple scale with higher qualities demonstrating better adherence); and behaviors of adherence and non-adherence.

Circulatory strain: BP was estimated multiple times at 1-to 2-minute spans, in a sitting situation following 5 minutes of rest. The mean sitting systolic blood pressure (MSSBP; from this point forward SBP) and diastolic pulse (MSDBP; from this point forward DBP). BP control was characterized per the 2007 ESH-ESC rules winning at the hour of the review: SBP < 140 mmHg and additionally DB < 90 mmHg, aside from patients with diabetes mellitus or potentially high or extremely high TCVR, in which case targets were <130/80 mmHg.9 The new 2009 reappraisal10 advocates < 140/90 mmHg focuses for all populaces, including diabetics, however as the examinations were directed under the ESH-ESC 2007 rules, we utilized the lower BP focuses for diabetic patients or patients with high or exceptionally high CV gamble in the examination.

TCVR (BSCORE and Great): TCVR was accounted for by doctors utilizing the SCORE cross-characterization of BP by risk factors (eg, smoking, dyslipidemia), metabolic disorder, diabetes, and laid out CV infection (MI, coronary supply route sickness, cardiovascular breakdown, cerebrovascular circumstances, fringe blood vessel illness) or renal sickness (characterized as serum creatinine > 1.5 mg/dL). Potential arrangements included: normal gamble - low added risk - moderate added risk - high added risk - extremely high added risk. We figured 'change in TCVR' by taking away gauge TCVR from follow-up TCVR, yielding potential scores from −4 (most prominent improvement in TCVR) to +4 (biggest deteriorating of TCVR). We likewise characterized patients dichotomously as appearing or not showing a decrease in that frame of mind no less than one class at 90 days. Patients with laid out CV or renal illness or patients at pattern in the normal gamble class were excluded from these last two estimations as they couldn't work on in the TCVR characterization.

Particular factual examinations notwithstanding broad rundown measurements, each study included progressed demonstrating methods to recognize determinants of BP values, TCVR change scores, BP control, and accomplishing a TCVR decrease of something like one classification.

Staggered or progressive direct displaying each taking part doctor enrolled a few patients; hence patients couldn't be viewed as free however rather 'settled' under their treating doctor. We accepted that the nj patients enlisted by the jth doctor could share some extent of fluctuation in BP values and TCVR change owing to their normal doctor, conceivably influencing the two factors preceding any understanding explicit factors. We applied genuine and contingent two-level progressive straight demonstrating. Genuine displaying measured the fluctuation in persistent results owing to a doctor class impact (intraclass connection coefficient [ICC]). In the contingent models BP and TCVR were first analyzed considering doctor level factors. The coefficients in this way inferred were utilized accordingly in the assessment of patient determinants of the BP and TCVR adequacy results.

Various leveled strategic relapse

This was utilized to show patient-and doctor level determinants of uncontrolled BP at 90 days; also, in the BSCORE and Brilliant examinations, to distinguish autonomous indicators of progress in TCVR.

We have introduced rundown insights from irregular impacts meta-investigations (Z measurement, Fences g, P worth) to assess impacts of BP decrease, considering between and inside concentrate on contrasts, and relationship among's pre-and post BP values. We have included match-matched measurements (McNemar's and Liddell's tests) to introduce the factual meaning of changes in BP control contrasted and pattern. We have introduced McNemar-Bowker's test to assist with evaluating the upgrades in TCVR (improvement in paired conveyances). Concerning ICCs, we present measurements from arbitrary impacts meta-examinations across review (Z measurement, P an incentive) for SBP and DBP, and χ2 for each review with TCVR (test against the invalid ICC of 0.00).

Results

In this segment, we audit the total discoveries across the different examinations for the viability results: BP values and control; as well as TCVR for the BSCORE and Superb examinations; the extent of difference in these viability results that is represented by a doctor class impact (Table 5); the staggered displaying of SBP, DBP, and TCVR; calculated displaying of uncontrolled SBP, DBP, joined SBP/DBP; what's more, accomplishing a decrease in TCVR of no less than one classification.

Viability results

Circulatory strain SBP and DBP values at benchmark and following 90 days of valsartan-driven treatment were comparative across the seven investigations. Utilizing weighted midpoints, SBP diminished from a mean (±SD) of 155.9 ± 15.4 mmHg to 137.5 ± 11.8 mmHg, while DBP diminished from 91.5 ± 9.6 mmHg to 82.0 ± 7.5. On the total, then, valsartan regimens were related with outright decreases in mean SBP of −18.4 mmHg (Z =−27.573; Supports g = 1.225, both P < 0.0001) and mean DBP of −9.5 mmHg (Z = −43.768; Fences g = 1.173, both P < 0.0001) contrasted and benchmark values.

All things considered, 38.2% had controlled SBP, 58.2% controlled DBP, and 32.0% controlled SBP and DBP joined at 90 days. In spite of the fact that BP control rates differed across our examinations, there were huge upgrades in extents of patients with controlled BP contrasted and gauge levels of control (all matched P < 0.001).

TCVR

By and large, across the BSCORE and Incredible investigations, patients' TCVR characterization diminished by −0.74 ± 0.95 class north of 90 days of antihypertensive treatment. At 90 days, around 60% of patients had a remaining TCVR that was no less than 1 classification lower than at standard. Really telling, maybe, are the noticed changes in risk classes from pattern to follow-up. As can be seen, whereas 45.9% of patients were categorized as having very high added risk or high added risk at baseline, this percentage decreased to 25.6% just 90 days later. Contrasted and standard, enhancements in TCVR were huge in both BSCORE and Superb (both McNemar-Bowker $\chi2 > 1000$; $P < 0.0001$). The modular subcohort of 42.0% with moderate added risk at gauge was diminished to 26.6% at follow-up, when low added risk turned into the modular subcohort (34.4%). At 90 days, close to half of patients (47.7%) qualified for the typical gamble and low added risk classifications.

Attribution of change to doctor class impact

On normal across the seven valsartan studies, 22% of the change in SBP ($Z = 22.954$; $P < 0.0001$) and 24% of the difference in DBP ($Z = 22.619$; $P < 0.0001$) at 90 days was owing to a doctor class impact. The typical change in leftover TCVR represented by a doctor class impact was 15% (BSCORE $\chi 2 = 87.48$; P < 0.0001: Superb $\chi 2 = 79.20$; P < 0.0001). Hence, anyplace from around one fifth to one fourth of patients' BP values following 90 days of valsartan-driven not entirely set in stone by the treating doctor - and this before any persistent factors entered the condition. Essentially, around one seventh of patients' adjustment of cardiovascular gamble was a component of the treating doctor.

Staggered demonstrating of circulatory strain values and TCVR

Through sum up the consequences of the staggered displaying of SBP, DBP, and change in TCVR following 90 days of treatment with valsartan-driven antihypertensive regimens in every one of the seven examinations. Following the noticed model capture, the top board records patient-and the base board doctor related factors that were held.

Systolic pulse Across the seven examinations, patient-related determinants of raised SBP (positive incline coefficient) included: age; SBP at the underlying conclusion of a patient's hypertension and SBP at beginning of a valsartan-driven treatment routine; risk factors like diabetes and retinopathy (as an intermediary of cutting edge diabetes), complete cholesterol at standard, and being a patient who fits the profile of being profoundly powerless against uncontrolled pulse. Patients' drug conduct was a reliable determinant. Nonadherence had a SBP-hoisting impact. Conversely, patient or potentially doctor evaluated adherence had a SBP-bringing down impact. Doctors who had been rehearsing longer would in general have patients with higher SBP levels toward the finish of 90 days. On the other hand, seeing more hypertensive patients was related with a diminishing in SBP; as was involving proof based systolic triggers for commencement or heightening of antihypertensive treatment.

Diastolic pulse Patient-related factors that had a DBP-hoisting impact included being male; DBP at introductory analysis and at inception of valsartan treatment; obesity; fitting the profile of high weakness to uncontrolled hypertension; also, longer time spans between pulse estimations. Nonadherence adversely affected DBP, yet adherence a beneficial outcome. Other DBP-bringing down factors included age, corresponding Pro inhibitor treatment. Similarly as with SBP, patients seeing more established doctors would in general have higher DBP, however doctor insight in treating hypertension had a DBP-bringing down impact. Involving diastolic triggers for therapy inception or increase, and regularly working out patients' generally cardiovascular gamble were additionally prescient of lower DBP.

TCVR

The translation of slant coefficients for the staggered models for changes in TCVR is something contrary to what applied to SBP and DBP. The purpose was to quantify improvement (and hence a diminishing) in TCVR, with the most ideal score being −4 and the most horrendously terrible score being +4. Consequently a positive slant coefficient shows that a given variable demolishes TCVR, while a negative coefficient signifies that a variable decreases and in this manner works on the patient's gamble. TCVR deteriorated the higher the SBP at beginning finding and at inception of valsartan treatment, and if the patient had diabetes or dyslipidemia. Conversely, being female and not having prior risk factors was related with upgrades in TCVR. The biggest impacts were noticed for patients' TCVR level at gauge; note the progressive, reliably expanding negative coefficients for each degree of added risk comparative with the typical gamble for the populace at large. With the exception of two evident dumbfounding doctor related factors, no doctor determinants were held.

Strategic demonstrating of determinants of uncontrolled pulse and accomplishing a TCVR decrease of something like one class.

SBP control The probability of uncontrolled SBP is an element of such persistent variables as age, SBP at the underlying determination of hypertension and at standard, diabetes, fitting the high weakness profile, being at high added or exceptionally high added TCVR, smoking, hypercholesterolemia, non-adherence, and months slipped by since last BP estimation. Alternately, uncontrolled SBP was more outlandish assuming the patient was male, had controlled SBP at standard (and consequently was begun on valsartan since earlier line of treatment was not endured), no prior conditions or hazard variables, and doctor evaluated adherence. On the doctor end, while years practically speaking was related with uncontrolled SBP, control was more probable assuming that the doctor knew the right BP focuses for non-diabetic patients and works on as per the suggested SBP limits for therapy inception and strengthening.

DBP control Uncontrolled

DBP was an element of the diastolic understanding when hypertension was analyzed, being diabetic or hefty, fitting the high-weakness profile, and being at moderate added, high added, or extremely high added TCVR at beginning of valsartan treatment, and treatment non-adherence. Expanding age, the shortfall of previous circumstances and chance elements, attending Expert inhibitor treatment, and doctor appraised adherence were prescient of controlled DBP. Whether a patient started valsartan treatment with controlled or uncontrolled DBP was related with comparing control status 90 days after the fact. While, once more, doctors' a long time practically speaking was prescient of uncontrolled DBP, a high volume of hypertensive patients over the a year going before the review, expanded recurrence of visits in the initial 3 months following the determination of hypertension, and rehearsing as per proof based DBP edges for therapy commencement and heightening were indicators of controlled DBP at 90 days.

Joined SBP/DBP control A few of the determinants of uncontrolled SBP or DBP likewise impacted the probability of both SBP and DBP being uncontrolled. On the patient end, negative determinants included: age, SBP at hypertension conclusion and at standard, diabetes, fitting the high-weakness profile, high added or exceptionally high added TCVR, earlier MI, hypercholesterolemia, and non-adherence conduct. Positive determinants comprised of: male orientation, no previous circumstances or hazard variables, and doctor evaluated adherence; notwithstanding SBP and DBP both taken care of at benchmark. Doctor wise, years practically speaking was related with uncontrolled SBP/DBP, while having seen more hypertension patients throughout the course of recent months, realizing the BP focuses for non-diabetic patients, and rehearsing as per SBP edges for therapy inception and strengthening made control of both SBP and DBP at follow-up more probable.

TCVR decrease by somewhere around one classification Patients were bound to diminish their TCVR by something like one classification if at pattern they were in the moderate added, high added, or exceptionally high added TCVR classes, had no prior conditions, and were seen by their doctor as being disciple. On the other hand, being more established, male, diabetic, and dyslipidemic made it doubtful for patients to diminish their TCVR by somewhere around one classification. Justifiably, the couple of patients who had both SBP and DBP controlled at benchmark were additionally less inclined to diminish their TCVR.

Conversation

Our examinations affirm that second-or later-line treatment with valsartan, in its various definitions, has major pharmacotherapeutic benefits in bringing down

BP and TCVR inside a 90-day time span in patients for whom earlier line treatment fizzled or was not endured. In all seven studies, these effects were observed with remarkable consistency across time, formulations, and diverse patient, physician, and setting populations. The real-world efficacy of valsartan-centric treatment plans is thus established by our research program's conceptual, methodological, and statistical consistency. Further, this pharmacotherapeutic benefit was demonstrated to be supplemented by changing, making due, or considering patient-and doctor level factors that might adversely affect BP and TCVR results; also, advancing those that might improve these results. As such, we can finish up rationally that valsartan is to be sure adequate in reality as its pharmacologic advantages were displayed to win in spite of the enormous heterogeneity in patients, clinicians, and treatment approaches contrasted with RCTs.

We saw that valsartan regimens were related with outright decreases in mean SBP of −18.4 mmHg and mean DBP of −9.5 mmHg contrasted and gauge values. In their meta-examination of 354 randomized preliminaries of BP-bringing down drugs, Regulation et al detailed BP decreases related with ARB medicines at the least accessible portion (eg, valsartan 80 mg), two times the most reduced accessible portion (eg, 160 mg), and in double mix treatment. For SBP these decreases were −10.3 mmHg, −12.3 mmHg, and −14.6 mmHg separately, well underneath the weighted normal of −18.4 mmHg in our examinations. Triple blend treatment was related with a decrease of −19.9 mmHg, somewhat better than the single and double treatments in our examinations. Moreover, in this meta-examination DBP decreases related with the least accessible portion, two times the most reduced accessible portion, and double mix treatment were −5.7 mmHg, −6.5 mmHg, and −7.3 mmHg, separately, contrasted and the weighted normal of −9.5 mmHg in our investigations. Once more, triple therapy had a slight advantage (10.7 mmHg).

BP control rates changed across our investigations, with later examinations moving towards lower control rates. This pattern can be made sense of promptly as a component of the regimens considered. After some time, our examinations included progressively more grounded definitions of single and mix treatments of different measurements of valsartan, starting with 80 mg, 160 mg, and 8 mg/12.5 mg HCTZ in the Review concentrate to the full supplements of valsartan in addition to HCTZ (BSCORE) or amlodipine (Astounding). Conceivably, our examinations advanced from 'regular' hypertensive patients requiring second-line treatment to progressively more challenging to-treat, in the event that not treatment-safe, patients as studies advanced over the long haul.

The noticed control rates are reason to worry for clinicians as they might demonstrate relentless helpful latency in hypertension the board: not increasing treatment when targets based on evidence are not met. Then again, the control rates in our review are actually normal for Europe. Involving similar boundaries as our examinations (140 mmHg/90 mmHg; 130 mmHg/80 mmHg if diabetic), the overall I-SEARCH partner concentrate on detailed generally speaking SBP, DBP, and joined SBP/DBP control paces of 25.2%, 42.5%, and 21.2%, separately. These rates were 17.5 percent, 35.5 percent, and 13.4 percent in the countries of Northern Europe, which included Belgium, Germany, Sweden, and Switzerland. Note that different examinations have proposed different topographical control rates (SBP/DBP joined) for periods simultaneous with our own, incorporating 50.1% in the US48 and 65.9% in Canada versus 27.1% in focal and eastern Europe50 and 28.0% in Britain. This uniqueness might be an element of contrasts in mindfulness and treatment across districts, however concentrate on plan contrasts might contribute similarly to such an extent. As our examinations utilized comfort alluded tests, the I-SEARCH review might be a preferred benchmark over a populace based concentrate on like NHANES in the US.48 In any case, all control rates checked on here are underneath the 75% hypertension control rate considered 'ideal'.

Decreases and changes in TCVR saw in our examinations were because of hypertension the executives just - perhaps an analysis of any cases about the noticed impacts on TCVR. Seemingly, there could rather be justification for clinical hopefulness, yet introductory: sufficient hypertension the executives in itself results in fundamentally lower leftover cardiovascular gamble, a finding we likewise saw in a new report on the immediate renin inhibitor aliskiren. One can guess what the outcomes would be of conjointly overseeing circulatory strain, glucose, lipids, stoutness, diet, movement, smoking, and liquor utilization in patients at different degrees of TCVR. The typical abatements in the frequency of stroke (35%-40%), coronary occasions (20%-25%), and congestive cardiovascular breakdown (half) related with antihypertensive treatment subsequently could rise assuming that more than one component of the TCVR condition is tended to clinically.

TCVR highlights the significance of patient contribution - from adherence to their recommended drug regimens to making the important way of life alterations. It has been proposed that providing patients with information regarding their global coronary risk may result in subsequent risk reductions. A new deliberate survey of 18 investigations reasoned that such data might build a patient's precision of seen risk and inspire those at moderate to high take a chance to begin treatment. Be that as it may, it was related with just −0.2% to −2% 10-year decreases in Framingham scores, and whether this was an element of patient information or the force of the going with mediations was muddled. On the off chance that patient information is without a doubt not power,54 the response might lie in utilizing this data to rouse patients into better taking care of oneself.

Staggered and calculated demonstrating

Our examinations were quick to evaluate the doctor class impact in antihypertensive treatment. The ramifications are critical. Numerically, SBP could be worked on by 22% and DBP by 24% assuming that any doctor impact were taken out. While honestly a hypothetical activity, the SBP weighted normal mean decrease of −18.4 mmHg could be stretched out to −23.6 mmHg, and the comparing DBP decrease of −9.5 mmHg to −12.5 mmHg. This makes one wonder with respect to what doctor related determinants should be addressed to diminish the variety among doctors. The staggered displaying results from our examinations give significant bits of knowledge in the connection between experience, information, and proof based practice.

Dumbfounding outcomes or intermediaries for clinical carefulness?

As summed up, a few patient factors were related with results that appeared to be illogical; for instance, presenting with additional risk factors or receiving additional antihypertensive treatment simultaneously. Likewise, doctor factors like more prominent information about hypertension, its administration overall and in unambiguous patient subgroups, distinguishing right BP targets, rule compatible practice, late proceeding with training in hypertension, and longer encounters with recently analyzed patients were measurably huge signs of treatment result. Apparently perplexing, these outcomes all point at - speculatively in any event - the significance of doctor consideration and ought to be thought of, we accept, intermediaries of clinical cautiousness.